SCENAR
FOR
BEGINNERS

DR PETA ZAFIR

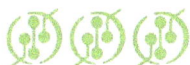

SCENAR
FOR
BEGINNERS

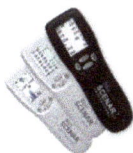

RITM SCENAR

DEDICATION

I dedicate this book to all those people past, present and future who through pain and sickness have found Scenar Technology and used it for regaining their health.

I thank RITM OKB ZAO, Russia for its development, RITM Australia for making it accessible for people in Australasia and for the trained, skilled and qualified professionals who use the true Russian RITM Scenar devices and technology, to assist clients every day in regaining strength, wellness and a pain free life.

COPYRIGHT

©2019 Peta Zafir
Peta Zafir Publishing
www.petazafir.com

ISBN 978-0-6452140-0-0

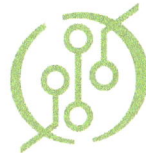

CONTENTS

DISCLOSURE

All comments made within this book are my opinions and experiences, taken also from the input of other experienced and trained SCENAR Practitioners, Teachers and Specialists.

I am not attempting to prescribe any medical procedures, it is my personal individual opinion and the information and Protocols mentioned in this book have been found by me, to be of use, in various conditions and situations.

However, this is not a medical book, this is a guideline of What I have done, Where I have placed Pads and SCENAR Devices, When I have treated, How I implemented Protocols and, Why I choose these actions and the results I gained personally.

I reiterate that all people are unique and individuals may have different results and that any course of action or changes that you undertake without the supervision of a licensed medical doctor, are at your discretion.

FOREWORD

I have written this book to make the use of SCENAR simplified and understandable. I do not go into a lot of Body terms and Physiology as some people know these and others don't. I make use of pictures and in some cases it is necessary to show the body physiology so you understand why placement and treatment are done, using a certain protocol or pattern.

Please be aware these are guidelines and if you follow them and find you go into an extended Healing crisis then speak to your professional SCENAR practitioner or trainer, as you may need to change your settings and frequencies to align with your unique condition or sensitivity.

There are many professional and Home SCENAR users that are confused about the What, Where, When, Why and How to use their new SCENAR Device.

It can appear overwhelming and you may become anxious and hesitant when faced with a chronic condition or an immediate accident; not know what to do or if your actions may exacerbate the issue.

The answer is very simple. The moment you place your SCENAR device onto the body there is change. Knowing **What** Settings to engage, **Where** to place pads or the device, **Which** protocols to implement and **How** to commence - this is what will speed the process up and give you information as to the next ongoing treatments. All these aspects combined give us the results for your personal body to change and recover.

I have in this book attempted to keep the information clear, precise and useable for all to benefit from.

CHAPTER 1 - FROM THE BEGINNING

In this chapter I will be clarifying what SCENAR means and extending your understanding of its procedures and functions. One needs to understand the meaning of the words used and how they are interpreted.

All this information gives a deeper understanding of the way the SCENAR works, its use to the person or animal, what is does and the outcomes you can expect.

SCENAR is an acronym for:

SC - Self-Controlled – a device which actively sends frequency impulses into the body via the skin and as a result of the skin's reaction, the frequency continues to constantly change and adapt.

EN - Energo-Neuro – the shape of the frequency impulse is similar to the body's own nerve signalling making it easy to be picked up by the afferent nerves, those nerves taking the messages to the brain and allowing the efferent nerves, those nerves carrying the message from the brain to utilise the information and make changes.

AR - Adaptive Regulator – when the device is placed on the body, the device adapts and changes its signal according to the body's reaction. As a result, every subsequent SCENAR impulse is different from the previous one.

It is important that you understand the guidelines for usage. These are set firstly by the Governmental bodies and also to make sure you don't deal with conditions that may create unnecessary outcomes.

These guidelines may differ in relation to your country's Medical Regulations.

The following contraindications are to prevent any reactions that you may not be able to work with. Therefore, you should not treat people who have:

- Individual intolerance
- Hyper sensitization
- Heart pacemaker
- Alcohol intoxication
- Acute infectious diseases
- Pregnant Woman

SCENAR can be used with and over Metallic implants - pins, plates, and screws; joint or hip replacements.

Do not work directly over inflamed veins or blood clots in the veins as they may create a situation where they become dislodged. When working with someone that has a lump, make sure the lump is checked or tested first before treating, as knowledge is power and there are different methods to use for different conditions.

If someone has wet or moist skin, wipe it down first before treating and understand that this can increase energy levels.

It is recommended to remove jewellery.

These indications indicate the health benefits that have been found to be valuable and positive:

- to analgesic therapies (Pain Relief) in pains in bones, muscles, joints and ligaments;
- to manage acute and chronic back pain;
- to treat primary dysmenorrhea;
- pain management after timed endometrial biopsy;

- to alleviate attacks and treatment of trigeminal neuralgia;

- to relieve pain in diabetic neuropathy (diabetic foot);

- to relieve pain in postherpetic neuralgia (Shingles) concurrently with antiviral drug therapy;

- to relieve pain in chronic/recurrent headaches and tension-related headaches.

When treating it is necessary for you to realise that the body may not change immediately however change is occurring.

Dr Hering Law of Cure states that Symptoms disappear in a certain order:

1. Reversal of Symptoms, the last symptom is the first to change

2. Symptoms move from the Top of the body downward – brain body connection

3. Symptoms move from more vital organs to less vital organs

4. Symptoms move from Interior of the body to Exterior - towards the skin; therefore, peripheral zones, such as Hands, fingers, feet and toes may take time to experience change

5. Chronic disease - takes about 1month for every year that the symptoms have been present

Chapter 2 - Let's Get Set Up

There are many ways in which you may decide to setup your device up. Some people like to hear the beeping which signals every 30 seconds and also when to change their battery. Some may also prefer to change their settings, utilising various Frequencies and Add-ons such as AM and Dose. Others users prefer no noise and favour the simplicity of pre-sets. Regardless of which way you work you Home SCENAR, it is necessary for you to know how to use all your features. This way you can also trouble shoot your device before needing interventions and repairs.

The Reset:

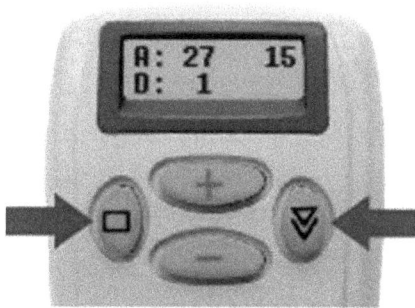

The RESET is the most important feature that assists in getting you out of trouble most times. This clears always all settings that you may have engaged, taking Energy to a low 1 and Frequency to 60Hz (Factory setup). Everything else is disengaged and turned off. Reset is also necessary after replacing the battery.

To implement a device reset simply hold both buttons for 3 seconds, then release - you will hear a series of beeps, indicating you have been successful.

Sound off or Sound On:

This is a way you can choose to personalise your device and it is done by:

Sound Off - press both the ⬇ and ➖ buttons together for 1second.

Sound ON - press both the ⬇ and ➕ buttons together for 1 second.

The Timer Feature (Sport D Only): allows you to implement more advanced protocol by recording the time in which the device takes to Dose. It is seen in the top right hand corner of the LCD screen and activates once placed on the skin. It will make a single beep every 30secs when in contact with the skin, achieving a maximum time of 9 min 59 sec, after which it will reset to zero and start again.

The following setting can be confusing for some and it may not be necessary for you to understand fully what they are at the moment, however it is important to understand what they do and how to use them.

F - Frequency indicating the number of stimuli entering the body per second, measured in Hertz (Hz), e.g. 15Hz means 15 stimuli hitting the body per second

FM - Frequency Modulation another frequency however this one works through a range of frequencies from 30Hz to 120Hz

E - Energy is the sensation you feel as you increase the power; that tingling feeling

AM - Amplitude modulation means it pulses on the skin - 3 second on and then stops for 1 second, on and off pulsing

D - Dose signals change in relation to reading the skin, delivering an individually measured dose according to the body's response. It is a more focused and individualized therapeutic effect and used for Point of Pain (POP), Local areas and treating Asymmetries

P – Preset – these are in the new Home Sport D devices.

P – Preset – these are in the newer Home Sport D devices.

New devices pre 2021 release have:

- P1 – Chronic conditions, combines AM + FM (30Hz – 120Hz). The FM in P1 preset is the same as FM on your device however in Preset 1, AM is added

- P2 – Acute conditions, combines bioGap & bioIntensity automatically relating to the skin reaction;

In the old Sport D+ the P1 utilized a FM modulation of 15-30Hz

Newer Home Devices Blue Case 2021:

- Dose 1 and 2 Modes

- 2 Presets - duration of each preset can be changed from 1min to 29 min, duration of each phase cannot be changed manually, each lasts 3 mins and can be used with the device built -in electrode, or any other electrode, including pads.

o   **P1 - ACU (Acute complaints) has 4 phases each lasting 3 mins:**

1.   BioGap, BioInt & Bio Frequency

2.   Low Frequency

3.   Medium Frequency

4.   High Frequency.

o   **P2 - SYS (Systemic complaints) chronic & vegetative conditions has 3 phases each lasting 3 mins:**

1. High Frequency
2. Medium Frequency
3. Low Frequency.Let's get started; here is my formula to start setting up your device

2018 and later Home Devices:

Choose a Frequency - 14Hz, 60Hz, 90Hz, 340Hz or FM or P1 or P2; notice these are all frequency settings

Increase Energy – this is a personal preference;

Then add AM or DOSE – and Dose may be used when the device is moving

Older Home Devices - DOSE or AM are not used when the device is moving:

Choose a Frequency - 14Hz, 60Hz, 90Hz, 340Hz or FM;

Increase Energy – this is a personal preference;

Add AM or DOSE – only if you are working on stationary positions.

Combinations permitted when you have engaged certain settings

Combi nation	Dose 1	Dose 2	AM	FM	F	P1	P2
Dose 1		✖	✓	✓	✓	✖	✖
Dose 2	✖		✓	✓	✓	✖	✖
AM	✓	✓		✓	✓	✖	✖
FM	✓	✓	✓		✖	✖	✖
F	✓	✓	✓	✖		✖	✖
P1	✖	✖	✖	✖	✖		✖
P2	✖	✖	✖	✖	✖	✖	

Understanding your device:

SCENAR Therapy treats the person not just a disease.

SCENAR Therapy treats the symptoms not a diagnosis.

A medical diagnosis of a condition or disease may assist us in understanding the processes of the disease and lead us to the areas and organs that may need to be avoided or treated, however the **Here and Now** *regime is still applied.*

The best results that I have found is when I change the settings on the device regularly, forcing a continual readaptation of the brain / body connection and creating dynamic change.

CHAPTER 3 - WHEN TO TREAT

The most daunting time when treating yourself or others is to take yourself away from your diagnosis or the name of your condition and look at what is occurring in the Body.

The Here and Now.

If you are not sure or there are no symptoms presenting, then you need to proceed with one of the general protocols. These include the 3 pathways and 6 points on the face, the Collar Zone, the Abdomen Zone or the Palm Zones, and you could also add the Informational Cleanse.

From these protocols you will be directed to where to go on the body for subsequent treatments, depending where the asymmetries show, pain areas are indicated and/or organ activation. Remember that these reactions are unique and very individual, so don't be worried if you find one person has more pain and another has less or another has pain activating where they don't remember any being there previously. This may be from an old injury or a clearing through the body as it follows Dr Herings Law of Cure - Top to Bottom, Inside to Out and Most important organ to the least important, Peripherals, Hands and Feet, Last.

The amount of time and frequency of treatments depends on whether the condition is chronic, acute, the client's age, state of health and their working and personal life. If they have time to rest, sleep and repair this is excellent, however many people are also trying to work, run a household, raise children and fulfil family responsibilities. I know you may ask: well if you are not well then none of those things matter, however financial and family tension can lead to more stress affecting emotional health.

As a general rule I do not treat longer than 20 to 30 mins, this will include a general protocol and possibly a Point of Pain (POP) treatment followed by a calming therapy to minimize a healing crisis. You can proceed for up to 45mins with pads, remembering to change the settings frequently.

Acute Pain is defined as having occurred within the last 2 weeks, or appearing suddenly, possibly as a result of an injury. You may need to use pads and treat every 2 hours or until you feel a reduction in the pain. Then reduce to a couple of times a day, then a few times a week until it is gone.

Chronic Pain has usually been experienced for many weeks, months or years and may be connected to an underlying condition. Treating Chronic pain too much may result in increased pain, however knowing the frequency that your body works well with can reduce this result. With chronic pain you may also find that the settings FM and Presets may antagonize your condition. If this happens replace these Frequencies with 340Hz and 90Hz and only add AM after you have been treating yourself for a few weeks.

CHAPTER 4 - WHERE TO TREAT

Treatment depends on many aspects, such as the presenting **Here and Now** condition. Sometimes you may not be able to access the area due to broken bones or severe burns being covered in bandages or plaster, if the area is highly sensitive, or you may have a reaction every time you treat it. I had one man who had broken his neck and was so highly sensitive in the neck zones, that when I placed the device in this area he would break out in hives and a rash. I proceeded to work on the reciprocal areas of the body, the lower back and lower abdomen. You can still work the body; you just need to understand where to go. I have put some reciprocal areas into this table to help direct you, as to where to go.

Pain / Complaint	Reciprocal Zone to
Face	Abdomen / Buttocks
Chin	Groin
Nose	Umbilicus
Ear	Flank (Torso)
Neck / Top of Spine	Sacral Spine
Elbow	Knee
Arm	Leg
Hand	Foot

23

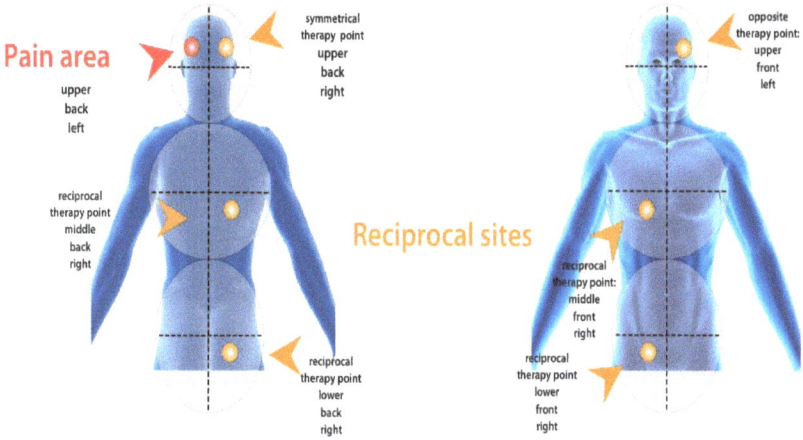

Pain area — upper back left

symmetrical therapy point upper back right

reciprocal therapy point middle back right

Reciprocal sites

reciprocal therapy point lower back right

opposite therapy point: upper front left

reciprocal therapy point: middle front right

reciprocal therapy point lower front right

While working on the body, you will need to be constantly scanning for any changes that may become visible, such as an asymmetry or small asymmetry.

Asymmetry's(AS) are signals on the skin that show where information blocks exist, places where the body is slow to adapt and repair; and therefore, this is where we need to work and create change.

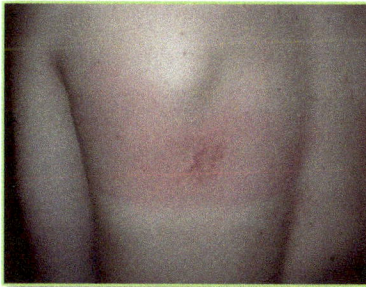

A large rectangular AS with a small interior red patch called a small asymmetry (SAS).

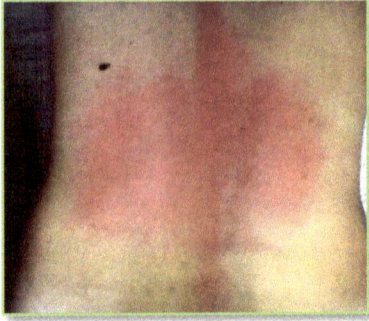

A large asymmetry (AS) with a small asymmetry (SAS) (pale strip) to the right of the spine and a pale roundish area at the right lower corner

Asymmetries (AS) can be seen as:

- Changes in the sound - as the device moves over areas, this can result in a larger clear sound or a muffled or silent sound;

- Change in colour - an AS is a red area or zone that becomes evident through treatment; a SAS is usually found inside a AS and is different t in colour, e.g. white area inside a larger red one. A SAS can also show as the reddest or the palest areas or the complete lack of colour;

- Change in sensation - high or low sensitivity of an area;

- Change in sound or concentration of pain in a small area or numb

- Change in Texture – becoming sticky or slippery or no traction on the skin

- When using Dose – SAS may be the Point of Dose and the Timer Reaction.

There are two modes of treatment we can implement - **Manual and Digital**.

1.   **Manual Mode** does not engage Dose and uses brushing techniques to find the AS; once found you will implement the 4 vector protocol or massaging techniques.

The 4 Vector Protocol is implemented when treating a small area, or where you know the point of pain (POP), also where there is an absence of a dynamic change, disturbance of energy flow, stable complaints and signs of small asymmetry. Also when you are working on small areas, such as the face, joints, buttocks, knees, elbows, over bruises, scars, spots, wounds, swelling and localised POP.

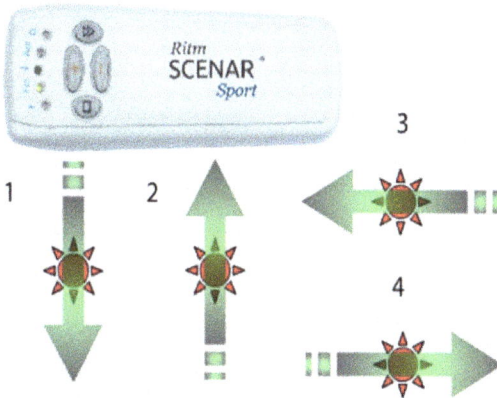

4 Vector Protocol:

- Work over the POP or AS;

- Brush from Top to Bottom, Bottom to Top, Left to Right and Right to Left;

- Brush each pathway 3 times. SCENAR likes to work in 3's;

- Find which direction shows the greatest resistance - more difficult to brush or sticky;
- Brush lightly and quickly in this direction 3 – 6 times, then repeat the 4 vector protocol again;
- Continue until you have Dynamic change – meaning it becomes less sticky or pain level has changed.

If there is still a POP, then change the setting on your device and proceed to massage this POP rotating your device on the POP in clockwise and anticlockwise directions.

2.   **Digital Mode uses Dose**. Take readings and record how long it takes to Dose; this information directs you to the next treatments. AS are the same as the Manual mode: change in sound, change in colour, change in sensation, and change in pain however we have the added information input of the Dose Reaction. Once you have located the AS treat it with Dose in each position for 2 minutes in a clockwise direction, or continue on this POP using Crosses, Galina's or General Protocols.

You will know when dynamic change has occurred by a change in pain, location of pain and/or change in mood. Remember that you or the person you are working on, may over the next 24 – 48 hrs experience a Healing Crisis. This can be where the pain may appear to become more intense and be experienced in different or more locations.

CHAPTER 5 – VARIETY OF LOCATIONS

A clear comprehension of Symmetrical and Opposite is necessary for awareness of pad placement. Symmetrical is the mirror image and Opposite is on the opposite side of the body. If POP is on the front of the body, the Opposite pad placement is directly behind on the back of the body.

Place one sticky pad on the POP and the other on the Symmetrical point; which means on the same side of the body and the same distance from the centre and treat these positions. Follow this by placing one sticky pad on the POP and the other on the Opposite point and treat these positions.

Settings: FM + Energy + AM - 20 mins, Change setting to: F 340Hz + Energy - 20 mins; next treatment you can swap the setting, start F 340Hz and change to FM.

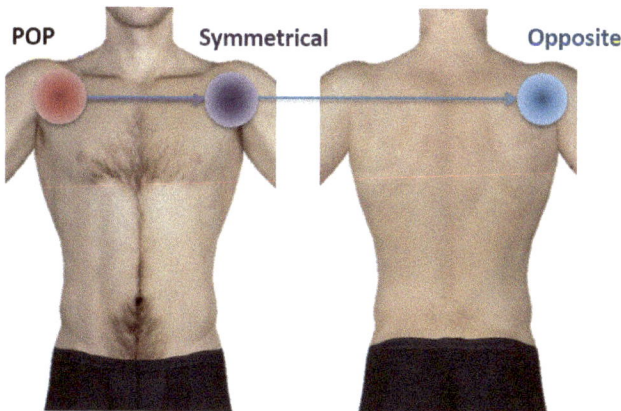

Horizontals are extremely useful and effective treatments - sometimes making a faster more beneficial change than treating for long periods over the same point. Mark you POP, go to the Opposite site on the spine; hold for 30secs and drag the device around the body passing over the POP, stop on the centre of the body; hold for 30secs continue to drag the device around the body back to the original **1st** position.

Setting: Repeat 3 times: F 90Hz: FM; F 340Hz; sometimes F 90Hz, F 340Hz and finish with FM may be more successful for some clients.

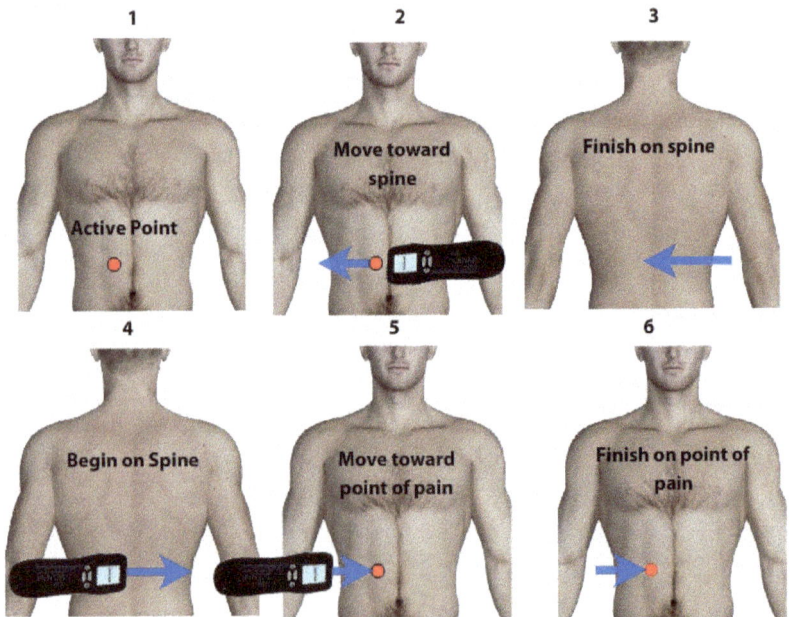

CHAPTER 6 - TREATING IN TWOS

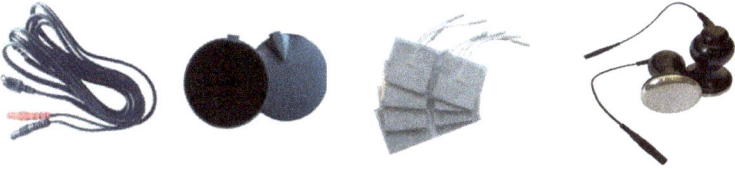

There are many times when it becomes advantageous to treat two positions on the body at the same time. This can be achieved easily using a 2-way lead attached to Sticky Pads, Carbon Pads or also using a SCENAR Paravertebral attachment.

The advantage of using pads is that they make treatment easy and accessible. It is important to understand that they do not replace the professional treatment or placing your device directly on the skin. It is a convenient and doable way to treat yourself when still active or resting. If you get the SCENAR Device onto your body it will make change.

Pads are also advisable when you need to treat any area that is difficult to reach, or you have no one else to assist treating you. Place the pads on the body (where to place will be explained in the next chapter), choose a setting and increase the power to a comfortable level for you.

Attach your pads to your 2 way leads and place one sticky pad on your POP and the other on the Symmetrical or Opposite position.

Do not remove or disconnect pads and 2 way leads by pulling the wire sections as this will damage your attachments, hold the thicker area to pull apart.

Small Cross Treatment

Small Cross must always be done in twos and the first cross is over the POP. It works well on bruises, spots, scars, swelling, across shoulders, up or down the spine, around knees and hips and for emotional treatments between the breasts and on the stomach.

Mark the first cross over the POP and follow the numbers in order. The second can be placed symmetrically, opposite, above and below or over the top of the first cross.
Setting: F 60Hz + Dose

Cross 1: Dose each position in order 1 to 5, and record the time it takes to Dose each point. On the point that has the shortest recorded time go back and reDose that point 3 times. Repeat for Cross 2

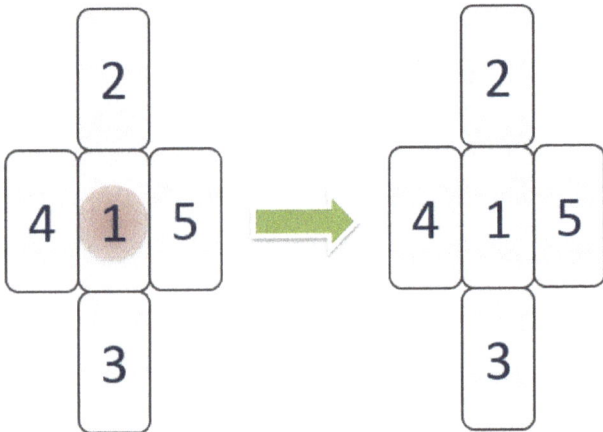

Galina Treatment

Galina's must always be done in twos and the first Galina is over the POP. It works well on bruises, spots, scars, swelling, on larger areas like the hips, buttocks, up or down the spine, on the stomach and with acute and chronic complaints.

Mark the first cross over the POP and follow the numbers in order. The second can be placed symmetrically, opposite, above and below or over the top of the first cross.

Setting: F 60Hz + Dose

Galina 1: Dose each position in order 1 to 9, and record the time it takes to Dose each point. On the point that has the shortest recorded time, go back and reDose that point 3 times. Repeat for Galina 2

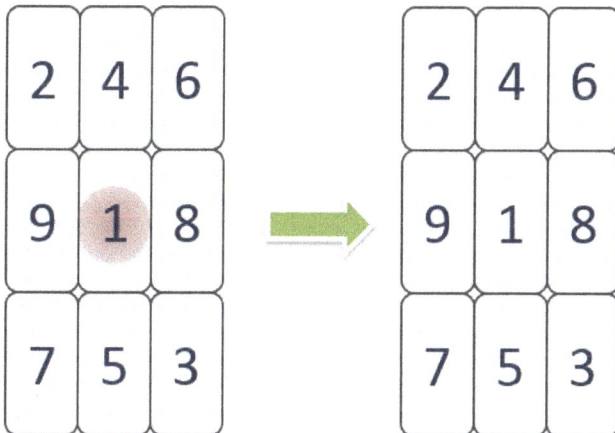

CHAPTER 7 – EMOTIONAL CONNECTION

The Autonomic Nervous System (ANS) is made up of two parts, the Sympathetic Nervous System (SNS) and Parasympathetic Nervous system (PNS) both originating from the spinal column. The SNS is stimulated for a person to speed up – Fight/Flight, and the PNS functions are intended to decelerate the body – Rest/Digest.

When prehistoric man faced a sabre tooth tiger attack, his body would prepare him to fight the animal or run away – fight/flight. Our bodies may be placed into the SNS when facing physical, emotional, psychological, mental and spiritual threats, injury, danger, trauma, chronic disease, and even simple daily activities such as work deadlines, phones ringing, family pressures and financial difficulties may activate this state. This reaction time is supposed to last 15 to 25 seconds allowing actions for survival to occur.

This involuntary action is intended to control the body response in times of stress and emergency by providing increased preparation. For these actions to occur several aspects of the body need to adapt. All of the organs start to prepare for the challenge it is facing, causing the muscles to contract; heart rate to increase, saliva production to reduce, digestive system to shut down and remain for an extended time which can result in advanced adrenal fatigue, chronic low energy levels, respiratory problems and decreased digestive and sexual function. Digestion and Hormones shut down because when you are at time of stress and danger you would not be eating, having sex or sleeping.

The PNS, the rest and digest state, can be initiated by having a SCENAR Treatment, starting a hobby, reading a book, taking a hot bath, petting your animals, joining in on social engagements, light exercise, grounding, gardening, walking in nature and techniques such as yoga, Tai Chi, Pilates, deep breathing, meditation and/or massage. When PNS is triggered it causes muscles to relax, heart rate to decrease, improved digestion as digestive enzymes are released, restores calm in the body, conserves energy and allows the body to rest, relax and repair.

Sympathetic Nervous System (SNS)	Parasympathetic Nervous System (PNS)
Go Go Go	Stop, Calm
Fight / Flight / Freeze Responses	Rest / Digest Responses
The body prepared to fight or take flight	The Body slows reduces and relaxes
Stress Response	Relax Response
Adrenal Glands activated	Repair & Growth; Balance & Homeostasis

A Fast reference understanding Fight / Flight & Rest / Digest processes

I have found in my time working with clients, that there is always an emotional component attached to every injury, accident, illness and health complaint. When a body believes it is under attack, it activates the SNS. Therefore, whenever you are treating Stress, Anxiety, Shock, Loss and Sleep Deprivation make sure you include one of the following protocols.

Setting:

1. Place pads on the SNN and C7

   - F 340Hz + Low Energy + AM

   - FM + Low Energy + AM

2. Pads on Sternum and Mid Thoracic

- F 90Hz + Low Energy + AM

- F340Hz + Low Energy + AM

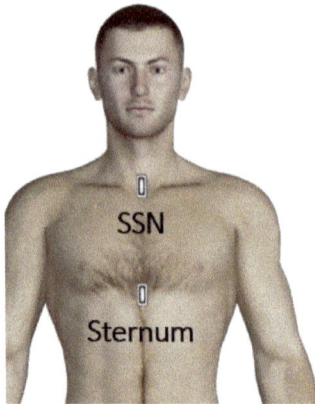

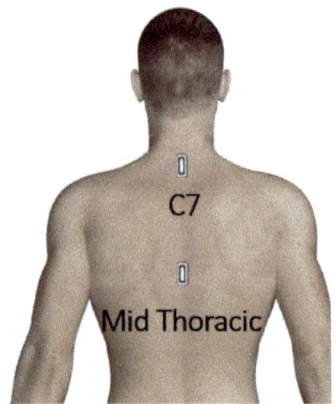

When working with emotional issues, and even physical issues you need to also treat the heart.

Setting:

- Treat with Crosses between the breasts – F 90Hz

- Pads - between breasts & what I call the Thoracic Heart, the opposite place on Spine

  - F 340Hz + gentle energy + AM – ½ hr

- Under Hairline on the top of the neck and the Coccyx F 60Hz

- Then move to SSN and C7 – F 340 or FM + Energy + AM

When working with Depression I have found the following protocol of great use:

Setting: FM, Working on the Spine, Start under the hairline, hold the device for 30secs then move down to the next position hold 30 secs. Make sure you overlap and do now leave gaps. You can work on the front on your body from SSN to Public Zone when working on yourself.

Work up the body to increase energy, and work down the body to relax.

Chapter 8 – Injury

When you have had an injury, involving trauma, sprains, strains, bruises and lacerations, it is important to start treatments as soon as possible. Inflammation will be triggered instantly, and scar tissue starts to form in a few days, so the sooner the better. Treating with your SCENAR will assist in accelerating the reduction of pain and swelling, promotes healing, speeds up the recovery process, increases the Range of Motion (ROM) and improves strength and performance.

I have had many clients who have gone in for knee surgery and commence treatment immediately after the operation, in the hospital. They have experienced less pain, had a aster recovery and a full range of movement in a shorter period of time.

When you have pain in a joint or along the arm and leg doing a Lymph Drainage Protocol may assist in increasing blood flow and activating the flow of the lymph system.

Lymph Drainage Treatment Setting:

- Arms - Treat each joint – Wrist, Elbow, Shoulder
- Legs – Treat each point – Ankle, behind Knee, Groin
- PADS - Place pads at each position, treat then move up
- DEVICE - Keep device in contact with the skin
- Circular Clockwise Motion
- P1, P2, FM or F340Hz + Energy - 2 – 4 mins on each point
- Longer if sticky or painful, then move to next point

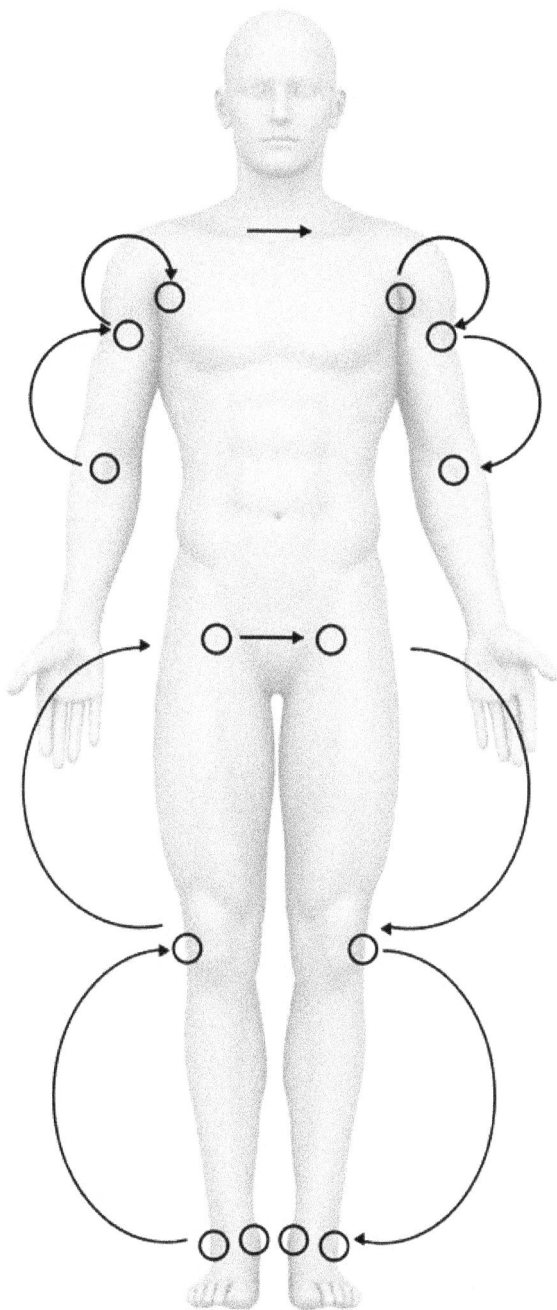

A guide to pain, its possible origins and treatment suggestions

Pain Type	Probable Body Structure Involved	Suggested Settings
Dull, Aching, Cramping	Muscle	Alternate F 60Hz and F340
Sharp, Needle-like, Tingling	Nerve	Alternate F 340Hz and F60Hz
Deep, Boring, Dull	Bone	Alternate F 14Hz and F90Hz
Sharp, Severe, Intolerable	Bone Fracture	Apply to opposite side to fracture. Acute pain 340Hz or Preset 2
Throbbing, Diffuse	Vascular	FM massage gently POP, if too painful apply to points around POP 30 sec each, Brush 4 Vector, apply every 2 hrs if needed, find asymmetry hold 5 min FM+AM, when finished brush over area F 340Hz

With neuropathic pain it is important to utilise both low and high frequencies, in order to activate, calm, stimulate then soothe; keep energy low. I have found high energy may increase an inflammatory response making the pain worse.

CHAPTER 9 - BACK AND SCIATIC PAIN

Many injuries and pain which may be caused by other conditions can be improved by treating two positions using pad placement.

Treatments for Back Pain Settings:

1. Pain on the back – Place the first pad on the POP and draw an imaginary horizontal line to the closest point on the Spine, place the second pad.

2. Pain throughout the Spine – Place a pad on the C7 vertebra and the sacral area of spine

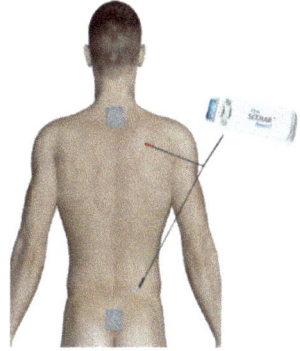

   Setting: FM + AM; Energy to comfortable; Treat ½ - 1 hr; Rest and Test - find new POP and move pads, Change to F 340Hz + AM. These frequencies can be interchanged using F 340 + Am first and finishing with FM.

3. Lower Back Pain – Place pads on both sides of bottom sacral zone and walk them up the lower spine.

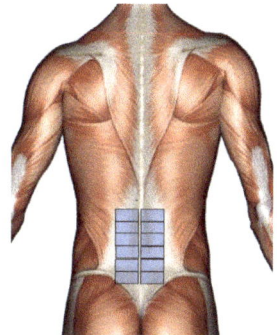

   Setting: F 340Hz + Dose; Dose each Pair, Change Pads moving up the spine and repeat. Record the time to Dose and FM for 2 minutes the points that took the highest and lowest time to Dose.

4. Sciatic Pain:
    - Compressions occurring at L4 (Lumbar) may create pain running form the lower back sometimes through the hips, the groin, through and around the knee and feet;
    - Compressions occurring at S1 (Sacral) may create pain radiating from the lower back down to the feet.

Setting: Place pads on the Lumbar or Sacral POP and the other on the POP on either the knee or feet - FM + AM; Energy to comfortable; Treat ½ - 1 hr;

Move the lower pad up to under the buttocks and F 340Hz + AM- ½ hr.

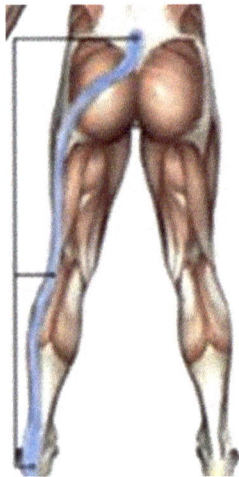

CHAPTER 10 - SHOULDER PAIN

I have found that shoulder pain can be derived from many areas and sometimes shoulder pain may be referred pain coming from other areas in the body, such as the front and back of the neck and the lower back.

There are several treatment protocols that you can work through:

1. POP and closest point on spine;

2. POP and Opposite point;

3. POP and under the armpit;

4. POP and SSN;

5. Dose clockwise around the shoulder – Record the Time to Dose –

- 1st treatment Dose the lowest time 3 times ;

- 2nd treatment Dose the highest Dose time 3 times;

- Alternate between highest and lowest times for Dose

6. Work horizontally from the Position on the spine outwards to the POP on the shoulder and return on the opposite side of the body; e.g. start at the back finish on the front of the body.

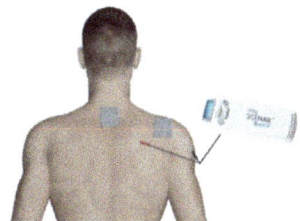

Setting:

- F 60Hz + energy;

- Treat 20mins; Test;

- Find new POP; Move pads;

- F 340Hz 10 mins;

- Test; Move pads;

- FM + Energy + AM – 20 mins.

CHAPTER 11 - KNEE PAIN

Knee Pain may occur as a result of a past or present sport injury or accident or a medical condition such as infections, gout or arthritis. The severity may vary from chronic or acute, location and severity and result in swelling and stiffness, weakness, feeling unsteady and limited ROM.

There are several treatment protocols that you can work through:

1. POP and closest point on spine;

2. POP and opposite side of the knee;

3. POP and behind the knee;

4. POP and under the foot;

5. Dose each position around the knee clockwise;

    a. Alternate between Dosing the lowest time and highest times points 3 times.

6. Work horizontally from Position on spine past POP, down under the foot, back up the other side of the leg, retuning and end in centre of the front of the body; e.g. start at the back finish in the front of the body.

Do a treatment each day and complete each setting for each treatment

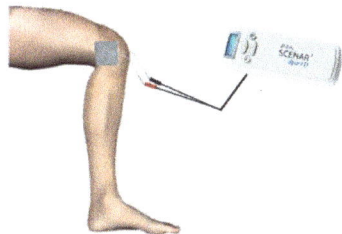

Settings:

- F60Hz + energy; Treat 20mins;

- Test, find new POP, move pads,

- F 340Hz 10 mins; move pads;

- FM + Energy + AM – 20 mins.

I have found when working with Muscle Tears, commence with FM + AM and finish with F340Hz.

You need to make sure you have dynamic change. This can be achieved by constantly changing your frequency setting, by adding and removing AM and DOSE settings, thereby creating a constant readapting and reassessment for the Nervous System and brain.

When I say constantly changing I mean one change in either Frequency, AM or Dose within one treatment.

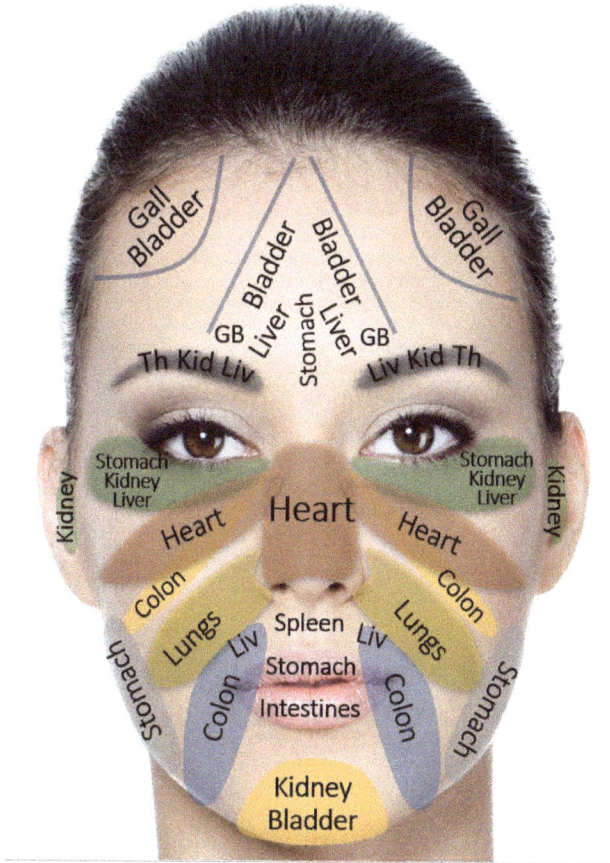

This picture shows you placement positions on the Face that relate to Body Organs. You can use this picture when looking for additional zones for treatment.

If you are finding that an issue is not making change then you may need to push the body by treating a point on the face relating to you complaint zone.

Settings:

- F 14Hz + Energy 20 mins then Finish on F 340 or FM 30 mins also;
- Dose each position three times.

Energy Points – Chakra flow

The Energy or Chakra points are specific areas where energy is emitted. When one has a physical, emotional, psychological, mental and/or spiritual stress, the body energy centres can shut down and restrict energy flow, thereby restricting and limiting repair and recovery. Treating these points is about treating your energetic body, allowing energy to flow and clear blockages, promoting a sense of balance and wellbeing.

Setting:

- 1st Day - FM + Comfortable Energy - 30 secs each spot;
- 2nd Day - Dose each spot

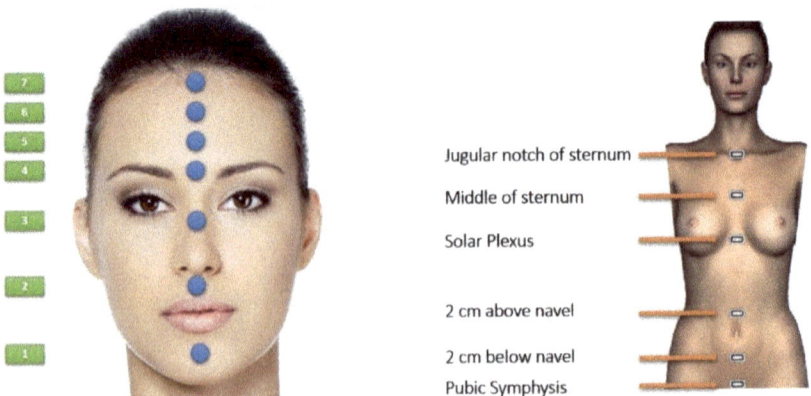

Jugular notch of sternum

Middle of sternum

Solar Plexus

2 cm above navel

2 cm below navel

Pubic Symphysis

Migraines

There is a difference between a migraine which is usually more intense and debilitating and a headache which causes pain in the head, face, or upper neck, and change in relation to frequency and intensity and

Migraines can be very personal and distinct for each person. They may result from a health condition, environmental toxins, food reaction or allergy, stomach disorder, nerve damage, medications, and hormonal changes such as menstruating or pre and post menopause. They can last for a few hours to days, range from acute to chronic, change in frequency, intensity and severity, and you may experience throbbing pain and/or a pulsing sensation. They can be usually felt predominantly on one side of the head more than another and often accompanied by nausea, vomiting, extreme light or sound sensitivity and vertigo. Migraines therefore, may make it necessary to treat several areas of the body to gain change and repair.

Settings if the migraine occurs:

- Front and Sinus - F 90Hz, High energy;

- Beginning of each eyebrow - Dose FM if fast, take Dose off and hold on this point for 2 mins;

- Cheek bone near nose - F90Hz + AM + Dose;

- Back of Neck – Gall Bladder & Urinary Bladder - F 90Hz, High energy - 2 mins then repeat FM for 1 min;

- Eyes – Liver - F90Hz + AM + Dose;

- Temples - F 340 - 2 mins each side.

Dental Pain

Settings - treating dental pain when you can identify the POP:

- Specific POP - can repeat every 2 hrs;

- Start POP then Opposite – F 340Hz - 2 – 3 mins each point;

- 4 vector – F 60Hz then treat asymmetries F 90Hz;

- POP - FM hold 1 min;

- Brush again – check for change;

- Repeat on opposite Point.

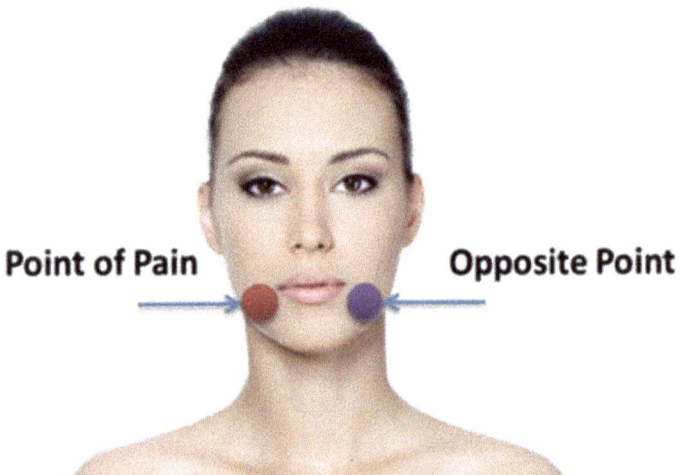

Point of Pain   Opposite Point

CHAPTER 13 – THE VAGUS NERVE

The Vagus Nerve is the longest cranial nerve connecting the centre of the brain to the whole body system. It is a Parasympathetic Nerve (PSN) affecting all areas of the body, stimulating the PSN System which involves heart rate, blood pressure, lungs, throat, controls sweating, toileting, saliva production, sexual arousal, improves gut/brain connection, abdomen, digestion, taste, speech, stress and anxiety and sends anti-inflammatory message to the body. The Vagus nerve may be overstimulated by conditions such as emotional and physical stressors and/or disease or surgery which in turn may result in feeling of vertigo.

I have found that when I work on and with the Vagus nerve, my clients have reported very good health changes; feeling more peaceful, less anxious and improvements in all organ function throughout the body.

Stimulating the Vagus nerve has been used for treating epilepsy, depression, bipolar and anxiety disorders and due to the anti-inflammatory actions of the Vagus nerve it may also assist in disease, such as rheumatoid arthritis, heart conditions, Crohn's disease, inflammation from diabetes, Parkinson's and Alzheimer's.

I always finish my treatment sessions by dosing from behind the ears, running down to the base of the neck; thereby activating the Vagus nerve. I use Paravertebral attachments however if you don't have these you can use small pads. I have found that all conditions effect the body by affecting the SNS which results in inflammation; by working the Vagus nerve you are assisting in reducing and eliminating this inflammation.

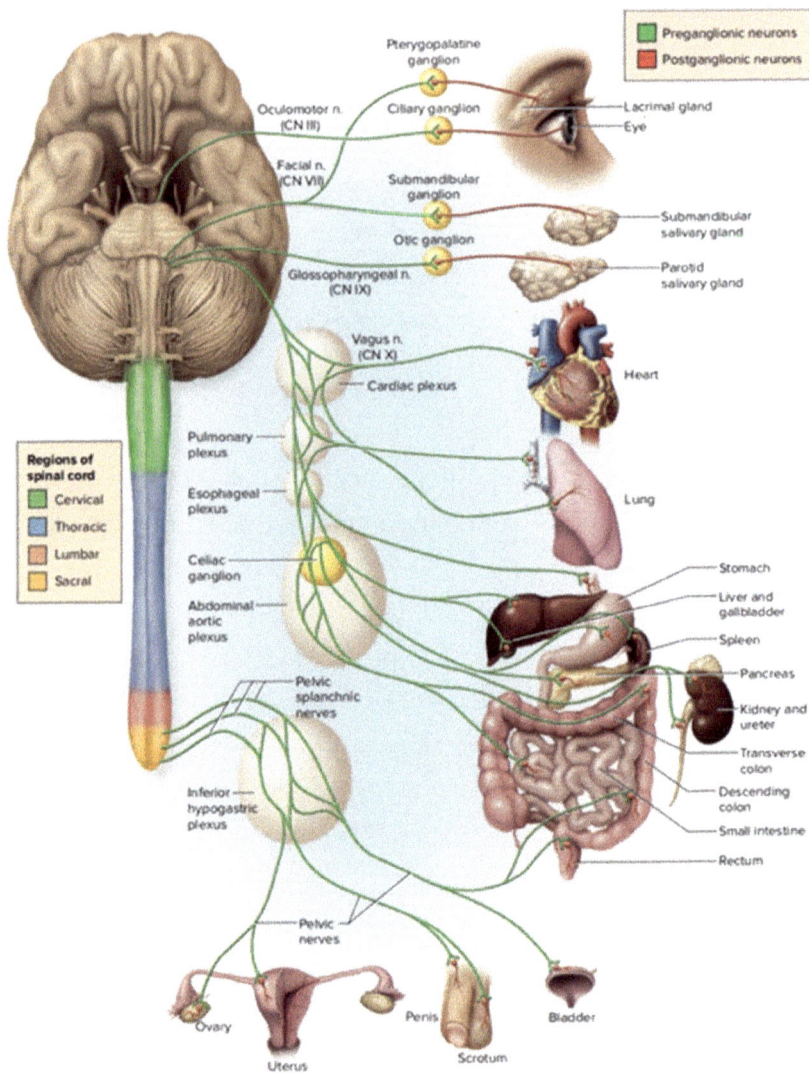

Pterygopalatine
ganglion

| | Preganglionic neurons |
| | Postganglionic neurons |

Oculomotor n.
(CN III)

Ciliary ganglion

Lacrimal gland

Eye

Facial n.
(CN VII)

Submandibular
ganglion

Otic ganglion

Submandibular
salivary gland

Glossopharyngeal n.
(CN IX)

Parotid
salivary gland

Vagus n.
(CN X)

Cardiac plexus

Heart

Pulmonary
plexus

Esophageal
plexus

Lung

**Regions of
spinal cord**

Cervical
Thoracic
Lumbar
Sacral

Celiac
ganglion

Abdominal
aortic
plexus

Stomach

Liver and
gallbladder

Spleen

Pancreas

Pelvic
splanchnic
nerves

Kidney and
ureter

Transverse
colon

Inferior
hypogastric
plexus

Descending
colon

Small intestine

Rectum

Pelvic
nerves

Ovary

Penis

Bladder

Uterus

Scrotum

CHAPTER 14 - 3 PATHWAYS AND 6 FACIAL POINTS

Trigeminal nerve pain may present as a severe, shooting pain or intermittent pain triggered by speaking, applying makeup or brushing your teeth. It travels from the face to the brain and may last for minutes, hours, weeks and longer. It may feel like an ache, a burning or cause spasms and the most affected areas being the teeth, jaw, lips, gums, cheeks, even eyes and forehead. It may focus on one side or over the entire face. It is more prevalent in woman than men and usually over 50 years old. Therefore it may be age related and can also be related to certain diseases such as Multiple Sclerosis, tumours, surgical injuries, stroke and facial trauma. In treating the 6 facial points you are also influencing the trigeminal nerve.

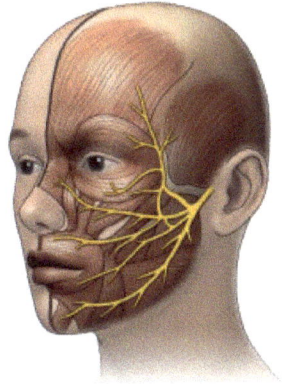

This protocol is found to assist in reducing pain, by supporting and influencing the body's adaptation process, to regulate the central (CNS) and autonomic nervous system which includes SNS and the PNS and also offers guidance for future treatments.

There are 2 protocols you can do, and time and severity of the condition may influence your choice.

BRUSHing is a faster treatment and may activate asymmetries, yet the skin and POP may be highly sensitive to brushing; DOSEing is specifically working more intensely on the POP and doesn't cause as much movement irritation.

Settings - if treating yourself

Protocol - 3 pathways and 6 points on the face

1. Central Path – Start on Suprasternal (SSN) - Hold 5secs, brush to base holding at the Public Bone for hold 5secs - Repeat 3 times
2. Repeat on your Right side if treating yourself, hold 5 secs to base hold 5 secs – repeat 3 times
   a. If treating someone else it will be on your Left looking at the person
3. Repeat on your Left side if treating yourself, hold 5 sec to base hold 5 secs – repeat 3 times
   a. If treating someone else it will be on your Left looking at the person
4. 6 points on the Face – reduce power – Dose each point
5. The Dose that has the lowest Dose time, Hold for 2 mins on that point using FM

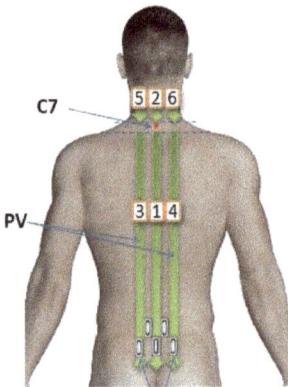

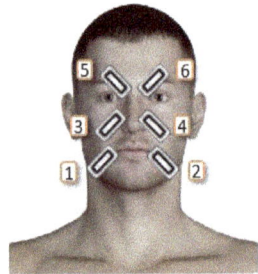

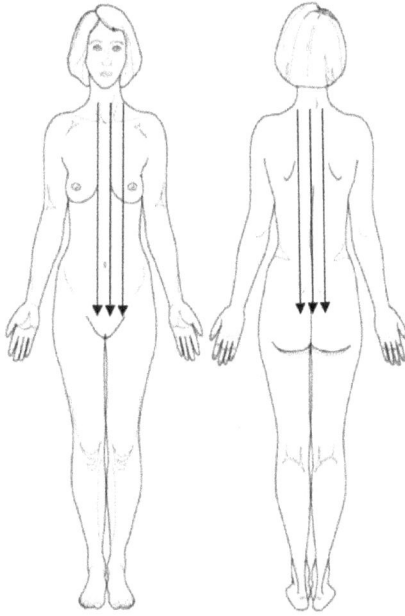

Dose

DOSEing gives a fuller, deeper and more accurate information as to where to treat, How to proceed and adds strongly to the adaption processes.

Setting:

3 pathways on the Front of the Body:

1.	Central Path below SSN - Dose each point from SSN to Pubic Bone; then above SSN

2.	Record the time for each Dose; Highest Dose time – Dose 3 times or FM for 2 mins.

3.	Repeat for the Left Pathway – below SSN then above, record highest Dose time.

4. Repeat for the Right Pathway – below SSN then above, record highest dose time.

5. Compare the highest Dose times for Right and Left Pathways and Dose the highest 3 times or FM 2 mins.

6. We always move from the centre point to the left and then the right, remembering that it is the practitioners left not yours. So if you working on the front of your body it will be your right and then left.

6 points on Face:

1. Reduce power – Dose each Point;

2. Highest Dose time - Dose 3 times or FM 2 mins.

3. The next time you treat Dose 3 times the lowest Dose Time

4. Change intermittently between Doseing the lowest time, and then the highest time.

If you are alone and unable to have someone treat your spine, then there are other positions you can self-treat to gain the benefits of this treatment. Understand that they also work the body however working directly on the spine is always the first choice.

Other placements on the body:

1. Front of the Body – SSN to Pubic Bone
2. 3 pathways on the hips at Front Hip
3. Down Leg from Groin to Kneecap
4. Down Arm – from inner wrist to elbow
5. Down Side of the body, running over the hip or upper body

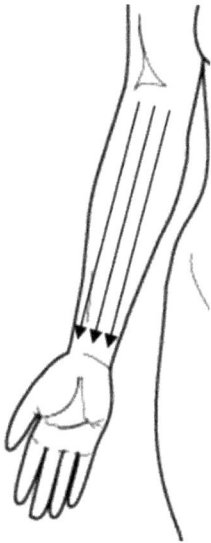

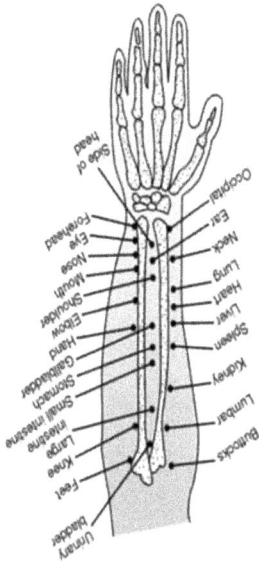

Side of head
Forehead
Eye
Nose
Mouth
Shoulder
Elbow
Hand
Gallbladder
Stomach
Small intestine
Large intestine
Knee
Feet
Urinary bladder

Occiput
Ear
Neck
Lung
Heart
Liver
Spleen
Kidney
Lumbar
Buttocks

Head, Ears		Eyes, Tongue
Teeth		Nose, Mouth
Throat		Neck, Shoulders
Thyroid Gland		Hands
Heart		Lungs, Breasts
Gallbladder		Liver
Stomach		Pancreas
Spleen		Adrenals Glands
Kidneys		Bladder
Small Intestine		Colon
Caecum		Sex Organs
Back		Feet

CHAPTER 15 – COLLAR ZONE BRUSH

The Collar Zone protocol may be advantageous when working with conditions relating to the Neck, Head, Shoulders, Arms, Hands, Emotional states and Immunity. Work from the hairline down and from the inside out to the shoulders making sure that each pathway touches or overlaps

Settings: alternate between these setting each time you repeat the Collar Protocol:

F 90Hz + Energy;   FM + Energy + AM;   F 340Hz + Energy + AM

Setting for Brush Collar: on the back of the neck

1. 5 secs at the top, drag down, stop at bottom of protocol, and hold for 5 secs

2. Repeat 3 times

3. Start on the left side, top to bottom, and middle of the neck going out towards the left shoulder

4. Repeat on the right side.

Setting for the Face: Reduce energy, brush bottom to top or Dose each point.

Setting for treating another person: Start from the inner eyebrow, work out to the left and then repeat on the right – this is facing your client.

Setting for treating yourself: Work from the inner eyebrow on the right and work outwards toward the right side of the head and then repeat on the left - repeat each path 3 times

Setting for treating the adrenals: Repeat 3 times; If no asymmetry, repeat in FM. If there is an asymmetry, do the 4 Vector protocol until change.

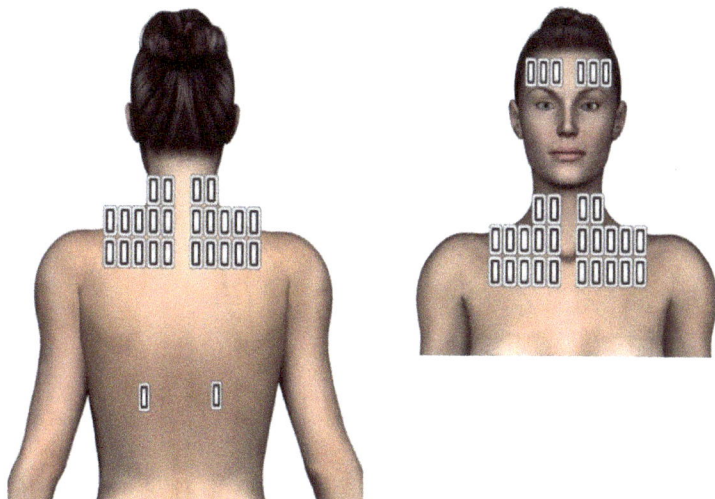

Repeat Protocol – Brushing and Next treatment - Dose each position;

Alternate - Highest Dose – Dose 3 times or FM hold for 2 mins; **Lowest Dose next time** - Dose 3 times or FM hold for 2 mins.

CHAPTER 16 – NECK RING OR PIROGOV RING

Neck Ring Protocol may benefit conditions relating to the Throat, Sinus, Allergies, Inflammation, Hormonal, difficulty in swallowing as seen in Multiple Sclerosis, and to boost the Immune System. It is a simple and fast yet very effective protocol. I have also found with headaches, not migraines, and some eye conditions (discussed in Chapter 19), this treatment can give relief by increasing blood flow and circulation to the head. Depending on the condition if I am trying to drain the head of mucus, throat pain etc. then I make my 1st ring high on the neck just under the jaw line, the 2nd ring slightly below this and the 3rd ring at the bottom of the neck. If wanting to increase energy, and blood flow to the head then I reverse this pattern. The 1st ring is low on the neck, the 2nd ring is above this and the 3rd ring is under the jaw.

Setting: F 60 Hz + Energy

1. Hold on back of neck vertically for 30 secs.

2. Drag slowly in a clockwise direction around the neck and stop when you arrive at the point of the neck you started from

3. Hold 30 secs

4. Then return in a anticlockwise direction back to the start point

5. Repeat 3 times

6. Remembering that one route clockwise and returning anti-clockwise is considered the first pathway

7. If there is an infection in the throat or neck start using F 30 or F 15

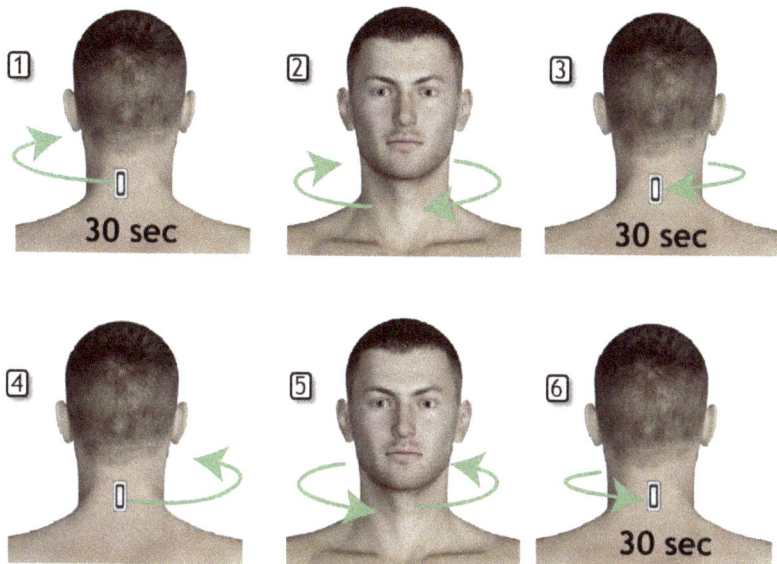

CHAPTER 17 – PALM ZONE

I have found this protocol to be very useful when working with conditions relating to Hormonal and Gynaecological Disorders, Urinary Systems, the Bowel, Prolapse, Prostate, Lower abdomen, Lower Back, Pelvic Pain and some types of Hip Pain.

Setting:

1. Brush each pathway 3 times or using Pads move two pads along the pathways placed one above the other

2. Front Pubic Area and Back Sacrum - FM + Energy + AM – 15mins using pad

3. 4 vector on any asymmetry that shows

4. Suprasternal Notch (SSN) and C7 - F 340Hz + Energy + AM – 30mins

5. 4 vector on any asymmetry that shows

Settings may differ depending on the conditions you are working with, this is where it is important to research and learn about the presenting complaint.

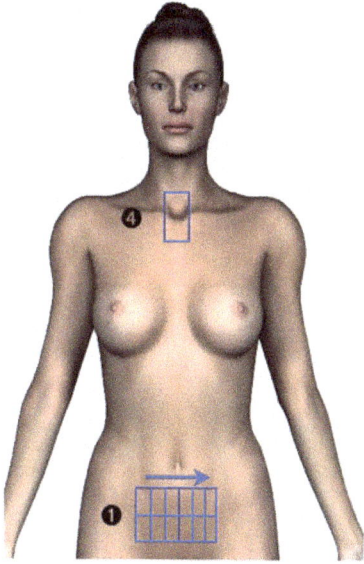
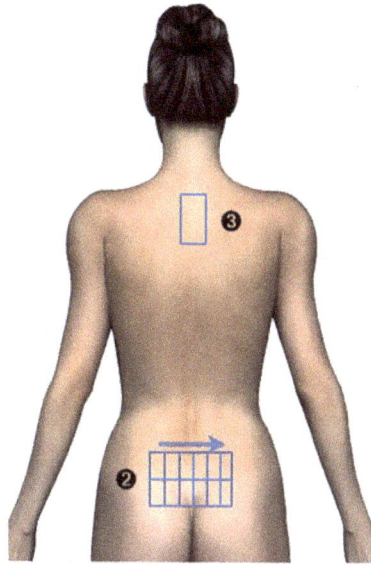

CHAPTER 18 - INFORMATION CLEANSE

This protocol can be used to quickly clean the body prior to a general protocol or you can complete the full informational cleanse as a way of rebooting the body's system. This protocol may influence changes in chronic pain, fatigue, sleep disturbance, increase energy, regulate the body's adaptive processes and place the body in a resting state.

Electrode is horizontal

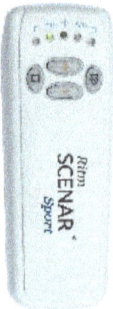

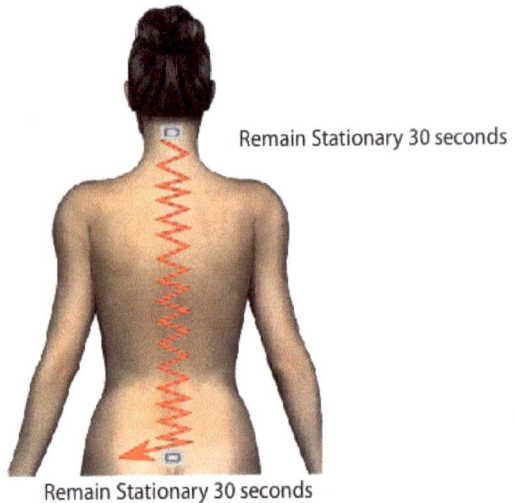

Remain Stationary 30 seconds

Remain Stationary 30 seconds

Setting:

1. For a rapid treatment hold at neckline for 30secs

2. Zigzag to the bottom of the pubic area and hold for 30 secs

3. Lift and go back to the top beginning point

4. Repeat 3 times

5. Change settings for each path: F 60Hz; F 90Hz; F 340Hz or FM

Setting for Full informational Cleanse:

 a. Hold device horizontally under hairline for 30 secs

 b. Slide back and forwards zigzagging across the spine moving down towards the coccyx

 c. Make sure the 3 pathways are all covered, it is better to overlap then have a gap

 d. Hold at coccyx horizontally for 30 sec

 e. Lift and go to the top and repeat

 f. Minimum of 3 times; Maximum of 8 times

  i. 1 to 3 pathways - 60Hz.

  ii. 4 to 5 pathways - 90Hz.

  iii. 6 to 8 pathways – FM / 340Hz.

 g. If you see an asymmetry show, then you can stop the protocol and treat the asymmetry with a 4 vector.

Setting for Alternate Information Cleanse:

Horizontally start at the point on the inside of the wrist and working zigzag to the elbow or from the SSN to Pubic Bone:

- Hold 30 secs at wrist or SSN

- Zigzag back and forward to the elbow or Pubic Bone

- Hold for 30 secs

- Lift return to beginning point

- Repeat 3 times

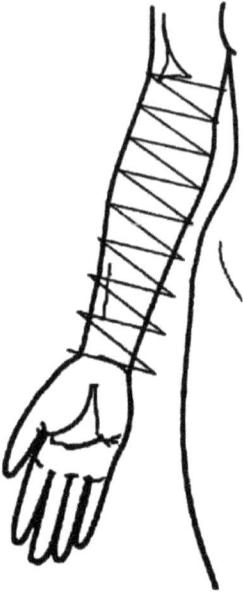
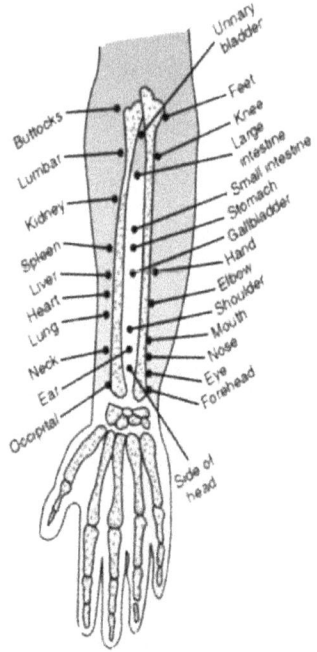

Urinary
bladder
Feet
Buttocks
Knee
Large
Lumbar
intestine
Small intestine
Kidney
Stomach
Gallbladder
Spleen
Hand
Liver
Elbow
Heart
Shoulder
Lung
Mouth
Neck
Nose
Ear
Eye
Occipital
Forehead
Side of
head

CHAPTER 19 – EYES

Brain Cross may be useful with insomnia, sleep disturbances, low energy, memory changes, sinus, stress, anxiety, headaches, migraines, depression, PMS, ADHD, addictions, vertigo, tinnitus, middle & inner ear disorders, vision, and poor blood circulation.

Setting: There are 3 positions to place pads:

1. Over or just inside ears – like an ear plug

2. F 60Hz + DOSE – if it doses too fast – leave for 2-3 min on FM

3. 7th Facial point and base of skull C1

4. F 90Hz + DOSE – if it doses too fast – leave for 2 - 3 min on FM

5. 6 pts on face – Dose each point

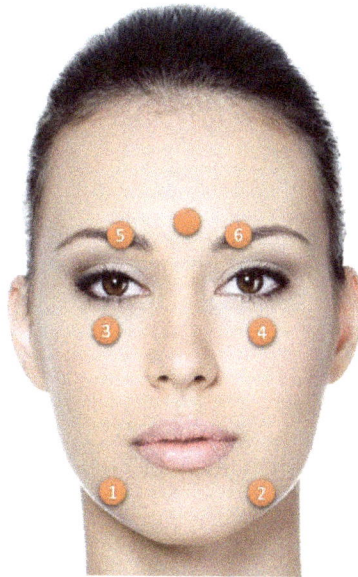

    a. Work in two - 1-2; 2-3; 3-4; 4-5; 5-6; 6-1; F 340Hz + DOSE.

Acute Eye Treatments

Acute eye issues usually occur from inflammation, injury or trauma. The eyelids need to be slightly open, look down and don't press hard. If you close the eyes, the eyeballs roll up and you only treat the top of the cornea, the eye's outer layer, covering the front of the eye and an important function in focusing vision.

Setting:

1. Work 7 points around eye

2. Dose each point F 60Hz or with pain F340Hz + AM; 1 mins each point

3. Finish with FM 1-2 mins on highest timed Dose

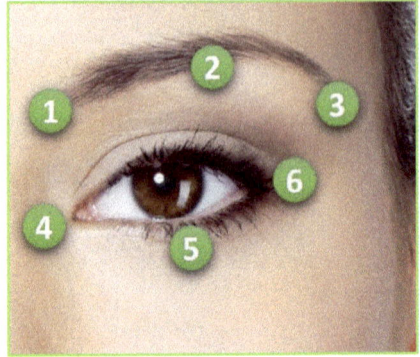

4. Next treatment use FM 1-2mins on the lowest timed Dose

5. Using the treatment protocol of 6 Pts on the Face

6. Treat only points 3, 4, 5, 6 pts – FM + AM for 5 min

7. 7th point between the eyes – 5 mins

8. Lymphatic areas - brush temples 3 times temples, front of ears & neck area

9. Repeat treatment 15-20 min per day

10. Treat both eyes; every 2 – 3 hrs with pain

Chronic Eye Treatment

Chronic eye conditions may relate to age-related or degenerative conditions such as cataracts, glaucoma and macular degeneration, and may be due to poor blood circulation.

1. Treatment needs to include brushing intensively on F 60Hz around the neck and shoulders – up and down briskly to get blood circulating;

2. Neck ring from base of the neck up to under the jaw – F 14 the repeat F 340

3. Hold at the base of skull – FM + AM for 3 – 5 mins;

4. Hold the positions front, back and below of ears – FM + AM – 2 mins each position;

5. 6 points on the face – F 14Hz - 1 mins each pt. or Dose each pt.;

6. Hold on the 7th pt. between eyebrows – F 340Hz - 3-5 mins.

If you find other areas start to become a focus, this is a good sign showing healing

Chapter 20 - Ear Treatments

This treatment may assist with deafness, tinnitus, hearing loss, temporomandibular joint (TMJ) pain and toothache

Settings:

1. Treating the armpits – FM + AM - hold 5 mins

2. Galina's on the hips - Dose1, F 15Hz + AM

3. Pads behind the Ear and back of the knee – FM + AM

4. Horizontal on the face, moving from the centre to the outer edge of the face – FM

5. 6 pts on the face – F 340Hz + Dose

CHAPTER 21 - TREATING CHILDREN

Always remember when treating children and animals that you need to have the energy low. Use a Frequency of F 60Hz as this will help to decrease the possibility of a healing crisis. The best areas to treat children are on the Abdomen and Spine. This may alter depending if they have come in for a particular condition, e.g. twisted an ankle or broken an arm.

Setting:

1. Abdomen

    a. Bush the whole abdomen from Left to Right, Top to Bottom and brush each path 3 times

2. Back

    a. Brush 3 pathways on the back start at the top and brush 3 times to the bottom of the spine

    b. 1st Centre, the Left and then Right side

3. Magic Hands

4. Pads on Feet and Hands

CHAPTER 22 – MAGIC HANDS

Treating the whole body can also be a way of getting dynamic change. Magic Hands is a treatment that you can implement while watching TV, or if someone can't present their back or front easily, and are sitting still. It affects the whole body system through the reflex energy pathways. Follow the pattern by number, remembering to always set your Energy level on the end of the fingers, as these are the most sensitive spot. Don't worry that you cannot feel it in the palm of the hand the signal is still going through.

Setting:

1. 1st Treatment

    a. Treat one hand with FM and the other with F 60 plus AM

    b. It doesn't matter which hand you choose with which setting

    c. Just remember your next treatment change them around

    d. Hold each point for 30 secs

2. 2nd Treatment:

    a. Set at F 90Hz

    b. Proceed to Dose each point

    c. Remembering to Dose the last point Number 17 three times.

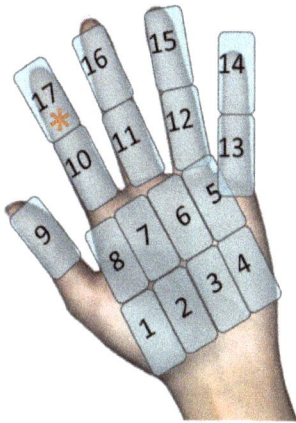
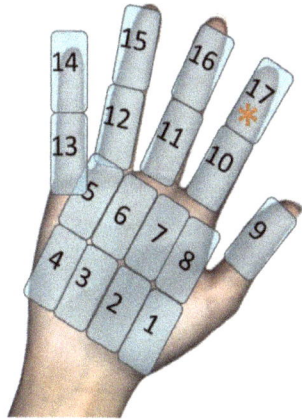

REFERENCE TABLES

Working with Combinations

Mode	Setting	Guideline for use
Energy Level	Low	When treating children, elderly and sensitive to electricity patients.
Energy level	Comfortable	Used for most patients.
Energy level	High	For acute pain.
Dose	1	When the painful area is similar in size to the device built-in electrode and to treat asymmetries.
Dose	2	For larger painful areas to quickly determine the location of asymmetries. Asymmetries should be additionally treated with Dose 1 or with brushing over the area.
Frequency	14Hz	Chronic pain, can also be used to sedate nervous pain – finish the treatment with higher frequencies.
Frequency	60Hz	Treating small muscles, Useful in cramping pain combined with AM. Useful in difficult pain complaints with no changes.
Frequency	90Hz	Ideal frequencies for general pain therapy.
Frequency	340Hz	Acute pain.
AM	ON	Acute or chronic pain with cramping.
FM	ON	Treat Asymmetries, pain without change, chronic pain.
Combination	14Hz + AM	Chronic pain with cramping.
Combination	60Hz + AM	Acute or chronic pain with cramping.
Combination	90Hz + AM	Acute or chronic pain with cramping.
Combination	340Hz + AM	Acute pain with cramping.
Preset 1	AM+FM	Treat Asymmetries, pain without change, chronic pain.
Preset 2	BioGap	Treat acute pain, pain without change.

Quick reference for Pain and Inflammation

Pain & Inflamation resulting from	Acute: Surgery, Injury, Dental, During Labour	Rehabilitation: Return to Normal activities	Chronic: More than 3 months
Device setting	Preset 2	Preset 2	Preset 1
	Frequency – 340Hz	Frequency – 60-90Hz	Frequency – 14Hz
	FM	FM	FM
	AM	AM	AM
	Stable Dose	Stable Labile Dose	Labile Dose
Energy Level	High	Comfortable	Comfortable
Treatment time	15-30min	45min	Up to 60 min

To maintain your warranty, your device can be repaired only by the manufacturer.

Clean the device on the outside thoroughly with alcohol wipes BEFORE and AFTER each use.

Problems:

- The device switches off during therapy there may be no skin contact

- The device switches off after 1 min – not good skin contact as the skin may be dry, not firm enough pressure or battery is empty or faulty.

- Repeated beep signal - replace the battery.

- No sound – is sound switched off

- Blank Screen, device freezes or cannot be switched ON - reset or

- Hard reset the device by placing the battery with opposite polarity for 2-3 seconds.

Warranty and Service

2 years from date of purchase - return to the manufacturer.

Warranty repair is not performed with broken warranty seals (inside battery area).

The device will be repaired at the expense of the owner in the following cases:

- the device was operated improperly
- the manufacturer's seals are broken

- the warranty period has expired

For all warranty and non-warranty repairs please contact:

RITM Australia Pty Ltd, PO Box 615, St Ives, NSW, 2075,

Tel +61 02 80114217;

Email: service@scenar.com.au

Peta Zafir Publishing

www.petazafir.com

Peta Zafir YouTube Channel

BOOKS BY PETA ZAFIR

Health in Poetry Book 1

Health in Poetry Book 2

Book of Sayings Book 1

Book of Sayings Book 2

Book of Sayings Book 3

Book of Sayings Book 4

Scenar For Beginners

All books are available in print and eBook format from:

www.petazafir.com/books

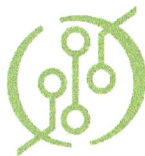

www.ingramcontent.com/pod-product-compliance
Lightning Source LLC
Chambersburg PA
CBHW041301040426
42334CB00028BA/3116